"180"

A "better you" exists, and you're only ONE decision away from becoming that person and truly living your best life! Here's my blueprint on how I turned my life around for the better and how you can too!

By

Mikey Bonasso

Table of Contents

Introduction

Hello, my friend! I am so excited for you to be a part of this quest for "better" with myself! Over the last several years, I have had the opportunity to experience a lot of amazing things, meet some incredible people, do some crazy once-in-a-lifetime type of stuff, and visit many beautiful places. I've had victories, triumphs, and home-runs but even more failures, setbacks, and strikeouts. I will say, however, at this point in my life, I thankfully don't have any regrets. I believe everything happens for a reason at the right moment. Had my circumstances been just a little bit different, this book may have never been written, and you wouldn't be sitting here reading it right now. Writing this book has been a goal of mine for the last several years, but I've always had some reason or excuse to put it off and wait for the "right time," which I realized there is no such thing. On this quest for "better," we must quickly realize that things don't just magically happen. If you genuinely want to improve your circumstances and start living the life that you know you're capable of having, we need to take the necessary action steps and put ourselves in a position to win. The player that hits the most home-runs spends a lot of time in the batter's box. You won't hit any homers from the dugout. There's never going to be a perfect time to take your at-bat, and there's never going to be a "perfect pitch." You just have to make the pitch perfect, make NOW the right time, and swing away! I finally said enough is enough; whether I feel I'm ready or not, I believe someone out there needs to hear my story, so I decided to grab my bat, swing for the fences, and hope my story leads you to some home-runs and victories in your personal life.

I'm by no means perfect, and even though I still consider myself a kid at times in many regards, I have had a lot of experiences in my short time here on this earth that I feel can bring massive value and impact many lives. You may be just a young millennial reading this, still in college just trying to figure out this thing called "life." You may be decades into a career that has been rewarding for you, but maybe not as fulfilling as it used to be. You may be retired and looking back on your life with gratitude, pride, or perhaps even regret. Regardless of where you are in this journey of life, my purpose today is to share with you some blueprints, strategies, tips, lessons learned, principles applied, and so much more to help you continue on your path; or maybe do a complete "180" if you're going down a road to nowhere (like I was) and know you need to change it immediately.

My prayer today is that this book will genuinely impact at least ONE life. Hopefully, much more, but if ONE person takes and applies these principles, changes their life for the better, and starts to impact and bless others, it will all be worth it.

Maybe that life will be yours, or perhaps someone you know… I THANK YOU again for your belief in me, the overwhelming love and support, and I hope this book finds you well and allows you to become a better version of yourself. Let's do this.

Chapter 1

Who Am I?

I believe it's safe to say at some point in our lives, we ask ourselves this very question: "Who am I?" It's a fair question; I mean, who doesn't want to know why we're all here, what is the meaning of life, and how do I fit into it all? You may be asking yourself these questions at this very moment, or maybe you have recently, which is maybe why you're reading this book right now. Maybe you're searching for answers and don't even really know the right questions to ask. I can tell you one thing, when you are aligned with your true purpose and mission, life is so much different. Every day has meaning. You're no longer just existing day-to-day and living for the weekends. You are designed to flourish and prosper. The purpose of writing this book is to share my journeys, struggles, failures, setbacks, and times of overcoming and triumph. Hopefully, this will help you answer some of these questions you've been asking yourself. Maybe even to do a complete "180" in your own life and turn from the things that don't serve you and begin to create a life of abundance that you deserve and are more than capable of achieving, whether you believe that or not. I believe that we are all called to serve and use our God-given talents and abilities to bless others. We all have unlimited untapped potential within us. Sadly, so many people will never even scratch the surface of what they're truly capable of. No one is perfect, and we'll never come close to it. But what if you could tap into just a small fraction of your fullest potential? What would life be like? Seriously, think about it. Because it's true and it's possible. But many will never take the chance. Maybe because of fear, uncertainty, not knowing what's behind the closed door... Maybe you're concerned about what your friends or family might think, or perhaps the fear of failing or the fear of succeeding (yes, that's a real thing). For a multitude of reasons, we miss out on life-changing opportunities every single day. Missing out on something isn't the end of the world, but we need to understand the deeper reason as to why we could have something so magnificent within our grasp, and we don't seize it because we're too afraid or maybe think we're undeserving or not good enough. If you never ask, the answer will always be "no," and I know from experience that life will pay you whatever price you ask of it. One powerful lesson I learned years ago was to DO IT SCARED. This means that it's okay to be afraid, but don't let fear stop you from moving forward and doing what you want, need, or are called to do! Understanding this valuable lesson is a game-changer. Don't allow fear to halt your progress and momentum. We all face fear at times in our lives, but the true champions acknowledge it, embrace it, and move forward anyway.

Before we can get into the necessary action steps to transforming into a better you, we must first acknowledge and recognize who YOU REALLY ARE to your core at this present moment. Understanding YOU and truly knowing YOU is critical. Self-awareness is key to becoming a better version of yourself. You must be real with yourself. This is when you look in the mirror and have some real-talk with yourself. Maybe your diet has gotten way off track, and you know you need to eat better, or lately, you've been binge-watching more Netflix than you probably should, maybe your bank account has a few less digits than you'd like to see, or your relationships aren't as healthy as they could be, or you're not as fulfilled at work like you used to be, or you're simply not happy. Here's what I can tell you; this part is not easy, but it's crucial and necessary. You can't begin to fix something if you don't first acknowledge that it's broken, temporarily. The good news is we can change ANYTHING; we can fix ANYTHING. "BETTER" awaits you. But you must first take a hard look in the mirror and face these things that you know need to be improved or maybe altogether eliminated. I want to be real and authentic with you, so I'll share some of my demons I've battled over the years. Since I was about 14 years old, I started to get very involved with physical fitness. I played sports all my life, and my freshman year of high school was when I began to get into weightlifting. It immediately became a passion of mine, even an obsession, and was something I did as a hobby, but also as a way to improve my athletic ability, and of course, make me look better for the ladies if I'm being completely truthful. In college, I wanted to bulk up and get as big and strong as I could. So, I naturally was consuming a lot more calories. I ended up starting a side-business selling workout plans, meal plans, supplements, and what I liked to call "healthy fast food" online, and I would usually work my business at night. I was consuming a lot more calories than usual, and many times at night, I would mix myself a cocktail, have some wine, or maybe a beer to relax as I worked on my business. Over time, this became a habit that I knew wasn't serving me well. I was getting stronger in the gym, but found myself weighing about 250 pounds at just shy of 6 feet tall; so needless to say, I was a pretty hefty boy for my height. Even though I considered my nights to be "productive," I almost always managed to get in my junk food, alcohol, and Netflix fix. I justified it for a long time, thinking it wasn't a big deal, and this is what most people do. I was trying to bulk up anyway so I figured the extra calories would do me good. At night, I was at least working, so I thought at least financially, I'm getting closer to my goals. But my health and physical state were getting worse even though I was in the gym every day. This was a case where I had to take a hard look in the mirror, realize that I wanted better for myself, recognize the areas I needed to work on, and then immediately got started. It was a process, but the decision to make the change happened in an instant. Although it was a decision I had already made, I had to reinforce it daily. But the moment of making the decision happened in a split second. Think about the word itself, "decision." The root word, "cision," comes from the Latin origin, meaning to literally "cut off." You are committing to something and "cutting off" all other options. Like the general told his army of soldiers, "If we want to take the island, we must burn the boats." Meaning there is no going back. We have made the decision and have drawn a line in the sand. Until this happens, you will never change, and your life will remain the same. If you truly want better, ask yourself, face yourself in the mirror, have that real-talk, then decide, and don't look back. Remember, nothing changes if nothing changes.

One of my mentors shared this story with me once, and I feel it's appropriate to share as I think it's what many of us deal with at some point in our lives. A man was walking through his neighborhood and heard an eerie, high-pitched squealing sound. Thinking it was just a bird or some kind of animal, he paid no attention to it. The next day on his walk, he heard it again. He was finally able to pinpoint where it was coming from. He went over to his neighbor's backyard and peaked over the fence and saw a dog sitting down and barking loudly. The man knocked on the door and the neighbor walked out. The man said, "Why is your dog barking like that? It sounds like he's in pain!" The neighbor said, "Well, you see, there's a sharp nail underneath him that he's sitting on." The man shook his head perplexed and naturally said, "Why doesn't the dog get up off the nail?" The neighbor replied, "I guess it's just not deep enough…" Many times, we are like the dog. The nail is there, and it's painful, but not painful enough for us to get up and move and take a new action. For many, that time to change will not happen until enough is enough; until you finally have that rock-bottom moment. I pray you don't have to experience that; if so, I pray it's not too "rocky." But many people have to go through what may seem like "hell on earth" before they finally make that change and make that decision. When enough is enough, when you're sick and tired of being sick and tired, you'll make the decision. And if you're not ready, maybe the nail isn't deep enough yet. Many people never get off the nail, and they live a life of pain and regret. "Better" exists. We are called to have life and have it abundantly. Don't settle, and don't allow the nail to win. Make the decision to get up off the nail, step into your better self, and truly begin to live your best life.

I had several rock-bottom moments. At least points in my life where I felt I was at an all-time low. I knew at that point in my life, I needed to make some physical changes ASAP. So, I started doing two things most people, including myself, hate doing; I started to diet and do cardio. I ended up losing about 20 pounds and got down to around 230. I looked so much better, was in much better shape, and actually on many of my lifts was much stronger. I was seeing results that became addicting and fueled me even more. Motion creates emotion. When you move, magic happens. Pushing a vehicle in neutral is hardest in the beginning, but once you have some momentum, it's smooth sailing. Momentum is powerful, in life, business, fitness, etc. I'll show you how to tap into personal momentum and pour gas on the fire, but we'll get into that later.

So, I get this crazy urge to do a bodybuilding competition. It was always something I talked about but never did, and I sure as heck didn't want to be one of those guys that always talked about something and never did it. So, I got my NPC card, submitted my application for a local show, and hired a coach. Little did I know how much work I had to do in a short amount of time. I only had 11 weeks to get myself in the best shape of my life. Looking back, it was probably the hardest thing I've ever done. Physically, it sucked if I'm being completely transparent. And mentally, you learn a lot about yourself and see what you're made of. When you're in a massive calorie deficit and severely carb-depleted, your brain starts to go a little nutty. I remember being extremely moody and even had a couple of nights I literally dreamed about pizza. No joke. Towards the end of my prep, I was working out seven days per week doing 60 minutes of fasted cardio on the stair-master usually around 5:30 in the morning every single day, then later in the afternoon would lift weights for an hour followed by another 60 minutes of cardio. About 3 hours of training, seven days per week. No cheat meals. No alcohol. No sugar. You get the idea. I was miserable. I was constantly sore and would take ice baths in the dead of winter, which didn't seem to help me much due to the excessive training and lack of calories. But it tested my mental fortitude like nothing else I had ever done before.

Going through that, I felt like I could do anything. And that's part of the reason I did it. I made a decision, and I stuck to it. It was a total "180" from my previous lifestyle. I don't share this at all to be boastful or with a "look at me" attitude. If you want to know the truth, in my division, I got 3rd place. Awesome, right? Here's the kicker; there were only three guys in my weight class. So yes, I got last place. The two guys that beat me, and deservingly so, were much bigger in all the right areas and better conditioned. But I weighed in at 197 pounds that morning. So last place or not, it was a massive personal victory for me. Fifty-three pounds down from my heaviest weight, and that's why I share this. It's about no one else but YOU. I didn't compete to win first place. I competed to see what I was really made of, to better myself, and test my potential. It was ME versus ME. You'll never know what you're capable of if you never get off the nail and TRY. Trust me on this; regret hurts so much more than failure. Failure's nothing. You get knocked down, but you get right back up and keep going. Regret is far worse. It's forever. It's permanent. Don't have any regrets. Get off the nail and step into your better self.

Okay, so you had some real-talk with yourself and recognized some areas that need to change, be improved, or altogether eliminated. When you're on a quest to improve yourself in any area, you need to eliminate what doesn't help you evolve. That may even mean changing up your environment, your friends and company you keep, and being very mindful of who you give your energy to. It's not to say to be a complete jerk and totally isolate yourself and become a hermit. But you do need to keep yourself "password protected" just like your phone, computer, or any other important files that you wouldn't want just anyone looking at. What I mean by this is you need to remove toxicity and negativity as much as possible from your life, and that may even be a close friend or relative. If it's someone you work with, live with, or honestly can't regularly avoid, love them and treat them like you'd want to be treated, but be mindful and don't allow their negative ways, views, and opinions to rub off on you or derail you from your vision and goals. You can love them and be their friend, but you don't have to hang out with them every night and adopt their lifestyle and viewpoints. You want to surround yourself as much as possible with people that are where you want to be in life. If someone has success in business, a wonderful marriage, a great personality and is full of positivity, or maybe a physique you desire to have, those are the types of people you want to seek out and befriend. Trust me on this; you will become the average of your closest friends. Be friends with everyone, and be kind always, but keep that inner circle tight because bad company can have incredibly destructive effects on your future plans and goals.

Many people that I have coached and mentored in the past may be able to recognize areas they need to improve upon. They may be able to identify a few friends or people in their life that aren't great examples for them and realize maybe time spent with them should be drastically limited. But a lot of people seem to struggle with a definite purpose for their life; the answers to questions such as, "Who am I? What is my purpose? And where am I headed?" This is something I battled with for years. Most of my twenties were an absolute roller-coaster. One positive thing is I tried A LOT of different experiences and ventures. I traveled a lot, met some amazing people, saw a lot, did a lot, and truly experienced more than many people do in a lifetime. But even though I experienced a lot, I was also all over the place mentally and never seemed to be in my "groove" and gift-zone. I knew what my passions were and what was fulfilling to me, but I felt like I didn't have any real direction and clarity on what my true calling was and what I was meant to do for the rest of my life, or at least then. They say if you chase too many rabbits, you'll catch none. That was me most of my twenties. I chased a lot of things and had some successes but many more failures. I felt like I had never really hit a "home-run" yet. But I knew I was just one more at-bat away. One thing that helped me tap into my passion, aside from being very self-aware as I discussed previously, was a series of questions I asked myself that I learned from my dad.

Ask yourself these three questions and write them down. "What do you love?" "What do you hate?" "What makes you weep?" By asking yourself these questions, you may grasp a much deeper understanding of yourself and what makes you tick. What makes you angry or sad? What makes you laugh? Asking yourself questions like these could lead you to something you are passionate about, or something that is fulfilling to you, or an area you can make an impact in for the lives of others. These questions will help you identify your "hot buttons." Maybe you can't stand bullying, or you hate to see people suffer; maybe you love animals, or you hate seeing children go hungry; you might have a soft spot for the homeless or veterans; you may hate to see people gripped with addiction or someone battling a disease or illness. I encourage you to take some time and ask yourself these questions. You may be able to learn something new about yourself, and this could set you on a path for doing not only something you care about that's fulfilling but also something that can genuinely make a positive difference in the world.

Chapter 2

A Winner's Routine

It's the offseason. A football player goes to
the stadium at 6 A.M. for an early morning workout
session. He sees a tall, thin white guy already there
getting in his workout. The player didn't know who
this guy was but admired his work ethic. The next
morning the player goes in at 5:30 A.M. and sees the
same guy in there already working out. He says to
himself, "Alright, tomorrow morning, I'll be here at
4:30 A.M. There's no way this guy is going to beat me
here." The next morning the player pulls up to the
stadium at 4:30 and sees the man sitting in his car. He
walks over to the man's car door, smiling and says, "I
guess we both got here at the same time today, huh?"
The man, covered in sweat, smiled and said,
"Actually, I just finished." That man was Tom Brady.

A man that was drafted in the 6th round with many people not having very high hopes for him, that ended up becoming arguably one of the greatest quarterbacks of all time. The point of this story is we aren't all born and blessed with crazy talents and freakish athletic ability like LeBron James. But we do have control over how hard we work. They say hard work beats talent when talent doesn't work hard. You don't have to be naturally gifted. It certainly helps, but it's not necessary. The goal is to go for it anyway and be willing to work your hardest for it. When I competed in my bodybuilding competition, I got 3rd place out of 3 guys. But I knew I gave it my all. I worked the hardest I could've possibly worked. Which is why it was a massive victory for myself. Now I'm certainly not saying you have to have a work ethic like Tom Brady to be successful in life or to become a better you. But what is important is that you start to develop a routine. The routine of a winner. Someone like Tom Brady, or Michael Jordan, or Tiger Woods, although very naturally talented, still had insane routines and work ethics that allowed them to become legendary in their respective sports. Routines that truly separated them from everyone else. If you can implement something new into your routine or a different behavior, within a few weeks, it will become a HABIT. I am a firm believer that success in business, sports, or anything in life comes from consistent behaviors and habits that bring you closer to your long-term goals a little bit each day. Habits will make you or break you. Literally. I can tell you right now, I've had some habits in my life, and things that I would frequently do that I knew were destructive and didn't serve me. So why do we do these things? A lot of times it's because it's convenient and it feels good. Maybe it's a release or a temporary escape.

In today's society, we want fast, and whatever feels the best and whatever is comfortable. We live in a "drive-thru" type world today. The word "comfortable" has become a bad word in my dictionary. I run from comfort. Comfort and boredom, at least for myself, is my kryptonite. Comfortable will make you broke, make you gain weight, make you unfulfilled, and lazy. Boredom will get you into trouble. It'll have you eating and drinking things that you probably shouldn't, perhaps even overindulging in them, and trying things to escape your reality. You want a reality that you don't need to escape from. How do you do that? It starts small. Very small. You brush your teeth every morning, right? I sure hope so. You probably hit that Starbucks drive-thru to grab your coffee every morning. Do you make sure to squeeze in at least one episode of that new Netflix series you just started every night? See, we all do things, little things, the same things, usually every single day. Why? Because it feels good. Because we enjoy it. Because it provides temporary satisfaction and is part of our daily routine. Maybe we just simply want to escape our life or our existing situation. I feel I can speak on this because I did this for years. A lot of what I'm saying right now is also me speaking to myself. To be honest, I still do it sometimes. But I've learned to control it. I don't let it control me. Not all of these things are negative by any means, but the point is to become aware of what your typical day looks like and how often you do the same things whether you consciously are aware of it or not. Also, why do we do these things? I used to hit a McDonald's or Dunkin Donuts drive-thru almost every morning, sometimes even a couple of times a day. I love coffee, but did I need a caffeine fix that often and that many times a day? Not really. But for whatever reason, I enjoyed grabbing a freshly brewed cup of Joe, and I did it regularly. It was convenient, and it made me feel good for that moment. I believe in balance. Netflix is great, but I like to earn it first. Meaning if I have a productive day or maybe I read ten pages of my book, for example, then I might watch something, but only after I EARN it.

We need to stop rewarding our unhealthy and unproductive behaviors. Go out with friends and watch a movie from time to time, but EARN it first. Before you splurge and eat an entire pizza in one sitting, go a few days of eating clean first. Use it as a reward for productive behavior, and it'll also give you something to look forward to. This is how you can slowly adopt new habits and eliminate bad ones. Focus on your daily behaviors, and once they become habits you do without thinking about, you are now on the road to a much better, healthier, and happier life long-term. Just like Tom Brady taking rep after rep after rep. Eventually, it becomes natural. Practice doesn't make perfect; it makes PERMANENT. So let's be mindful of what we "practice" daily. A massive tip I learned from another one of my mentors is called the B.U.I.L.D. system. It's a daily accountability system that tracks your activities, goals, and habits and makes sure that you're on the right path every single day. The "B" stands for "body." What is a physical goal that you can do every day, or at least a few times a week? Maybe it's a full-body workout or maybe just a walk around the block.

Focus on working your physical body multiple times a week, and I promise you, not only will you feel so much better, but you'll look better too! And you'll be amazed at how much more productive you are in other areas when you have those endorphins flowing! The "U" stands for "YOU TIME." Do something for yourself, every day. Maybe you like to golf, or go for a walk, read, meditate, or do yoga. Whatever that is for you, do it every day. Spend some time alone and getting in touch with your real self. This will not only help you create stronger self-awareness, but will give you better peace of mind, and will also strengthen the creativity side of your brain. The "I" stands for "income." Focus on income-producing activities frequently, whether it's for your job, business, side-hustle, or all of the above. After all, we are after "better" in all areas, right? The "L" stands for "relationships." Focus daily on your existing relationships, how you can improve them, and always be present in the moment. Eliminate distractions when you are around friends, family, co-workers, or whoever it may be and learn to be present and absorb every moment and memory because these are times and moments that we will never get back. The "D" stands for "development," which is your time to improve and invest in yourself; maybe read a book, take a course, seek mentorship, anything that's going to help you elevate your game. I try to B.U.I.L.D. every single day. You will have days where you may miss certain elements of this, but overall if you can implement this system into your daily life, you'll begin to see massive positive changes almost immediately.

Another important element to understand is the art and foundation of 'learning." I'm going to share with you a powerful secret that a very successful entrepreneur and mentor of mine taught me years ago. Once we become conscious and aware of these four elements, you truly can reprogram your brain and begin to learn new skills and habits that serve you. They are the four levels of learning, and these apply to literally everything. They are Unconscious

Incompetence, Conscious Incompetence, Conscious Competence, Unconscious Competence. Big words and may sound confusing, I know, but to put it very simply, I'll give you a real-life example of each. Most people that have a cell phone most likely have an iPhone or an Android. But if you went to a third-world country, for example, and showed a young child your smartphone, they may not have any idea what it is or how to use it. They are Unconsciously Incompetent on using a smartphone because they've never seen one before and have no mental reference-point of what it is or how it works. This is the first level of learning. The next level is Conscious Incompetence, which means that you are aware that you don't know how to do something. You may know what a piano is, but may not know how to play it and are aware that you don't know how to play it.

The third level is Conscious Competence, which is when you have learned the skill, but it isn't second-nature to you yet. Maybe the first time you rode a bike or learned to drive a car. You knew how to do it, but you always had to think about what you were doing when you were doing it. The fourth level is true mastery, Unconscious Competence. This is when you have learned a skill so well that you can do it as if on auto-pilot. Brushing your teeth or tying your shoes or even driving a car are some examples. These are things you can do without giving it much thought because you've done them so many times already, the muscle and cognitive memory are already there. Successful people understand these four levels and know if you can tap into that fourth level, you'll be unstoppable. So how do you get to that fourth level? Well, first, you have to TRY. Then it's all about practice and repetition and getting those reps in daily! I took a sales job in Richmond, Virginia, a couple of years ago, for a construction company that specialized in storm-restoration insurance claims.

To get our leads, we would go through neighborhoods and literally cold-knock doors. I remember the first time I got a door slammed in my face. Definitely not the most fun experience. But how I learned and how I started setting appointments was, first, I TRIED. I worked up the courage to knock that door, and in the beginning, I didn't even know what to say. I had somewhat of a script, but many times I would just "wing it." I had been in sales before, so I at least knew some basic principles of how to read people and body language and how to communicate with them briefly before they cussed me out and slammed the door in my face. Well, not too often, but that did happen many times. But how I got better was I just kept doing it. Each time adjusting my pitch and learning from each previous experience. I knew what separated me from being a rookie to being very successful in this industry was just a matter of TIME and REPS. This is encouraging news because this means that no matter how crazy or far-fetched or out of reach your goals or dreams may seem, they're just a matter of time and reps away. Anything can be achieved. You just have to have the courage to start and get your reps in, and I can tell you this from experience, you're not always going to "feel like it." But you have to learn to discipline those feelings. There were many times I did not want to knock doors and get rejected. But I knew with each door-slam, I was that much closer to a sale. There are days where the last thing I want to do is go to the gym. But I made a commitment to myself long ago to do something active and physical every day. I've never regretted a workout, but many times I've regretted not going when I knew I should've. You're not always going to feel like it, and if you're waiting for that spark of motivation before you take action on something, you're not going to be very productive long-term. Motivation is temporary. We must learn to discipline ourselves to take the necessary action regardless of how we feel. One thing I started to incorporate into my routine is taking a cold shower in the morning. I'm talking an ice-cold freezing shower.

I'll be honest; I hate it. It sucks. But I do it every day. I personally try to seek discomfort every single day. A cold shower is one of those things.

There are many health benefits to doing this, but I also do it to push myself through my mental barriers. I do it to prove to myself that I am in control of my body and my thoughts, and that's why I try to deny the flesh every day. This could be a cold shower or abstaining from something that you like to indulge in. When you sacrifice your flesh of things it wants, it makes you stronger in other areas, especially mentally. One of the best things I could've done for myself was doing that bodybuilding competition. I denied my body junk food, sugar, alcohol, parties, and late nights and replaced it with healthy food and many hours in the gym every day. That took some mental willpower. But I feel it made me stronger in the process. What is something that you indulge in maybe more often than you should? It could be food, alcohol, TV, or anything that doesn't make you better. Sure, it might feel good and be fun. But remember, we're on a quest for BETTER, and if that's truly what you want, we must discipline our fleshly desires and replace them with better habits and behaviors, which first starts by TRYING, and then getting in those daily reps!

Chapter 3

Your Greatest Wealth

Many people that achieve great financial success in life a lot of times sacrifice and neglect their health in the process, and then spend a lot of their wealth trying to get their health back. The real wealth is having your health. We've already talked about this a little and discussed denying your flesh and starting to develop better habits in your life and eliminating those that don't serve you. But in this chapter, I want to dive more into your overall health, not just physical but also mental, emotional, spiritual, and relational as well. In the previous chapter, we talked about developing a "winner's routine." I'm going to give you a few of my tips and secrets of things I do to optimize myself and perform at my peak. Some of these things you may never do and may not see the point in doing them, but I want to share with you what I do, why I do it, and how I feel it has helped make a positive impact in my life.

We talked about sacrificing your flesh and seeking discomfort daily, which is why I like to start my mornings with a cold shower. It wakes me up and makes me more alert, it tightens and tones your skin making you look younger, it helps blood flow and circulation, is great for cognitive brain function, and also helps sore muscles recover quicker. There's a reason many professional stars and athletes take cold showers and ice baths, not just for the physical benefits of it but also what it will do to you mentally. Another morning tip is I like to sleep with my blinds and curtains open. Now, if I wake up before the sun is up, then this doesn't apply, but usually, whenever the sun rises, I want that to be the first light I see. Most of us sleep with our phone by our bed, and the blue light from the screen can make you more tired and feel sluggish.

So, before I look at my phone in the morning, I like to take in that natural sunlight. Vitamin D is key! Self-care is critical. As I'm writing this, we're currently in quarantine due to the COVID-19 global pandemic, and I feel this time has made us all much more aware of the importance of simply taking better care of ourselves. You only get one body and one life. Having goals and big dreams is great, but it doesn't matter if you're doing destructive things to your body daily. Be mindful of not only how you treat others but how you treat yourself. There's nothing wrong with enjoying a pizza on Friday night or going out for some beers with friends, but remember, you're not a garbage disposal, so be aware of what you're putting into your body daily. Fill your body with foods that will optimize your daily performance and make you feel and look better. Let food be your medicine. A friend of mine that is a nutritionist and doctor once told me that most people don't actually know what it feels like to truly feel good. Think about that for a second. When she told me this, I had to pause and thought to myself, "Wow, that is so true!" Most people don't know what it feels like to operate at a higher level and feel good and not feel like crap every day!

Most days, do you feel sluggish and not your best and would rather just take a nap than do anything physical? We all have days like that, and it's good to have "lazy days" every once in a while. I am a big advocate of having balance in life. But how many days per week do you feel more crappy than alive, vibrant, and alert? We all have yucky days, but there's no reason that you shouldn't have 27-29 days of every month where you truly feel great! A lot of what I have shared with you so far is mental. But you are what you eat, and if you really want to maximize your potential, and prolong your days and years of your life, you need to make sure that you're doing the basics of taking care of yourself. Eat clean at least 80% of the time, drink lots of water, get good sleep, and be somewhat active. It really is that simple, and this is something that anyone can do and maintain. It's not some crazy routine, fad diet, or intense workout regimen. It's simply taking it one day at a time, eating clean most of the time, drinking water, and moving your body every day. Just by doing this, you can add years onto your life and look and feel so much better in the process. I believe if you want to have a happy, long, fulfilled life, your physical health plays a huge role. Just by simply being active and moving releases endorphins that make you happy. I aim to do something active every single day where I break a sweat and get my heart-rate up.

My physical fitness journey has helped me in so many ways, in so many different areas. If you're serious about truly bettering yourself, you cannot neglect the physical aspect of your health. Physical fitness for myself has not only helped me to look and feel better, but it has strengthened me so much mentally and has shown me a glimpse of how amazing the human body really is and how far I can push myself. The only limits are in our own minds. When you think you can't go any further, you can't do one more rep or run one more step, your body is only halfway done, but your brain is saying you can't do anymore. Physical training has been a great way for me to push past mental barriers and limits and see what I'm made of; when you feel you can't do any more reps, but then push to get one more, then one more, then one more. It truly is a mental war-zone, but just know you are far more capable than even you may believe. It makes me think of the 1997 NBA Finals when Michael Jordan had the flu, and no one knew if he was even going to be able to play. He ended up having a game that is still talked about today, hitting a 3-pointer in the final minute to seal the victory, and finishing with 38 points. Obviously, he was not a normal human and a legendary freak of an athlete, but overcoming that and doing what he did was a massive mental battle. He could've easily sat that game out and rested, but he ignored the pain and all the mental thoughts going on in his head, saying that he shouldn't be doing this and should instead be resting and hydrating. But he pushed past the mental barriers and physical pain and ended up having a legendary, iconic performance. We may not be as talented as MJ, but we possess the same mental power to push past barriers, fear, uncertainty, and doubt to get to that other side where all our goals, dreams, and aspirations await us.

A key component to your overall health is your mental health. It's crucial to keep your mind active and engaged and not allow it to get lazy. I'm a big movie buff, and as someone that is beginning to step into the entertainment industry myself, I do enjoy watching movies or shows as "homework" and "research." What I mean by that is I study the actors and actresses, their body language, how and why they act and react the way do, and so on. My point is I love to watch movies, and I'm not ashamed to admit that. But as you can see, it's something about myself that I identified and recognized and know that it can be a dangerous thing if I allow it to control me. For example, if I spend countless hours or days on end binge-watching movies or shows, that obviously is not healthy. But after a long, productive day to relax and watch an episode or movie is perfectly fine. I like to watch something at night because it allows my brain to shut down slowly and I can usually rest better. If I'm up late working or reading something, sometimes I will get super inspired or motivated, and it interferes with my sleep schedule. Again, this has been years of trial and error for me and understanding how I am and using that to keep me productive and allowing me to have balance in my life. That's why self-awareness and truly understanding yourself to your core is so important. It's okay to be "normal" and enjoy movies, or pizza, or ice cream, or beer, or TV. There's nothing wrong with these things, but understand that they can overtake you and quickly control you. Then they become habits and addictions that you feel you need every day.

For the longest time, I would avoid watching shows on Netflix because I knew I would be wrapped up in it and want to watch the entire season in one sitting. So, I would just watch a movie instead because, in less than 2 hours, it's over. I do watch shows sometimes now, but I've become more disciplined not to allow myself to overindulge. My best advice is to find your balance. Identify how you are and why you're like that, and then you can begin to develop a routine that supports that lifestyle. If I have a productive day, it's a lot easier for me to justify watching a movie that night. If I have been eating clean for five days straight, I'm probably going to reward myself with that pizza and ice cream. So the good news is you can have an everyday life with normal desires, but if you can learn to control them and use them as rewards for healthier habits, this is how you can see success in all areas of your life over time and have a healthy balance.

Chapter 4

Bulletproof Mindset

Your mind is an extremely powerful force. It's believed that we only use a small percentage of our brain's total capacity. I truly believe one of the most determining factors between someone that becomes massively successful in life versus someone that just lives an average life is their thoughts. I call this the "6-inch battlefield," and it refers to the 6 inches between your ears; in other words, your brain. I call it a battlefield because our brain is designed to keep us safe. That is why when something is uncertain, or there is a chance for failure or rejection, our brains want us to run from it because it views it as something that can be potentially "harmful" to us. But the crazy thing is, the lifestyle, the body, or the wildest dreams that we desire are on the other side of this mental barrier. Once you recognize and understand this, you can take action to overcome it. But if you're not aware of this, you will always be a prisoner to your fear and doubts. They may not even be your doubts but doubts that others have placed in your head that you now believe to be true. No one knows you better than you. So be very careful taking advice from others, especially if they are not where you want to be in life. Beware of the naked man that offers you the shirt off his back. People can't lead you to where they've never even been themselves, and they can't give you something that they don't have. You probably wouldn't take relationship advice from your aunt that's been divorced six times, or take nutrition advice from your cousin that is 120 pounds overweight. You get the idea. Protect your mind from doubt, especially if it's placed there by someone else.

Self-doubt is sabotaging enough; you don't need others' negative opinions on top of that as well.

Self-doubt and fear will destroy more dreams than anything. The main difference between the successful man that "makes it" compared to the man that lives an average life of unfulfilled dreams and endless regrets, is simply the successful man tries and doesn't allow the doubt and fear to win. I truly believe success is a state of mind. Which is great news because that means anyone can achieve it! You just have to overcome your doubts and disbelief. That's why I call it a battlefield. It's okay to be afraid. But don't let fear stop you from taking action. Do it scared! That's one of the best pieces of advice I can give you today. Be afraid, but take action anyway; eventually, you'll realize fear is just an illusion, and it's only your brain trying to "protect" you. F.E.A.R. can stand for False Evidence Appearing Real or Face Everything and Rise!

When I was working in Richmond, there were many times I was afraid to knock on someone's door. Especially in the beginning, when I didn't know what I was doing, what to say, and how to answer simple questions and combat objections. This is something that really helped me, even when I would make cold calls in my network marketing business, and that was the "1, 2, 3, GO!" rule. If you think about something too long, your brain will eventually talk you out of doing something. I remember when I was a young kid jumping off the diving board into the deep end at my grandparent's pool. My dad was floating in the deep end, waiting to catch me, and what seemed like a hundred times, I would run to the edge of the diving board and stop. My brain was telling me this may not be a great idea. What if my floaties don't work? What if I go under and can't get back up? This happens to all of us at many points in our life. When I would make a cold call or knock on a door, I would use this strategy. Take a deep breath, don't think about anything, then count to 3 and just GO! You have to take those 3 seconds and allow your brain to "shut off." Don't think, just act. And once you've taken the leap off the diving board and you're in mid-air, you realize there is no going back. Then after the fact you see there was nothing to be afraid of in the first place, and you realize that your fear was just a fake lie.

Your mindset is everything; it can make or break you. I truly believe thoughts are things. Be very careful what you focus your thoughts on and how you speak to yourself because you are always listening! If you tell yourself you're not good enough and that you'll never make it, your brain will believe that to be true. If you tell yourself you can't, you're right. But the same is true if you tell yourself you CAN. Just like in the beginning of time when God created the heavens and the earth. He said, "Let there be light," and there was! He literally spoke things into existence, and we possess that same power. If you can see it in your mind, you can hold it in your hand. Don't underestimate the power of your thoughts. They will form your reality. You may have heard of the phrase "the law of attraction," especially if you've read the book "Think and Grow Rich." I believe the "law of action" is far more important; however, I do believe that you can attract positive things into your life by being and thinking positively. The same is also true for negative thinking. One of my favorite quotes is, "life is always happening FOR us, not TO us." Let that sink in. If you can shift your way of thinking and accept this philosophy, your life immediately changes for the better. It's not easy, especially in the beginning, and it'll never be perfect. But once you're aware of this, you'll begin to notice a drastic positive shift in your life.

It's easy to complain when you're driving through town and seem to hit every red light. But what you don't see is that red light may have stopped you from getting into an accident. That's what I mean when I say life is happening FOR us, not TO us. Life happening TO us is a victim mentality. Life happening FOR us is the belief that everything that happens in our lives, good or bad, is for our ultimate benefit. You may not see it in the present moment, but that's where faith comes in. I've learned this lesson many times. Our plans may not always go the way we want, but for those that have faith, you know you're a part of a bigger plan that we may not be able to see yet. You just have to trust that all things will work together for good for those that believe. This is why having an attitude of gratitude is so important. You can't be mad and grateful at the same time. Those two emotions can't coexist. The more grateful you are, the happier you will be. Trust me on this. Every morning when I wake up, the first thing I say is, "thank you, God, for another day." It immediately puts me in a state of gratitude, which makes me happy and sets the tone for my day. If you're ever in an angry or sad mood, write down some things you're grateful for.

Once you do this, you realize how blessed you truly are and realize things could always be worse. You can also set reminders on your phone. There are a couple of different apps you can use. A few times a day, remind yourself to simply pause and just say "thank you" to God. I also use phone reminders a few times a day to pull up my goals so that I am forced to see them multiple times a day. Out of sight, out of mind. So put them in sight! I also set my reminders to inspirational songs that I like. Music can be a powerful tool and can instantly change your state.

Have you ever heard a song that maybe you hadn't heard in years, and it immediately reminded you of your childhood or made you think of a specific place or person? Music has a powerful effect on the mind, so I use songs that trigger specific emotions for me and use them as my notification sounds for my phone reminders. Seeing your goals in front of you while listening to a certain song you love can have extremely positive influences on your daily actions.

Remember the word "B.A.R." It's an acronym for Belief, Action, Results. It all starts in your mind. Your beliefs determine your actions, which determine your results. If you want different results in your life, you first must change your thoughts and belief system. This is why whoever you surround yourself with and what you allow into your mind has such a powerful effect. Whether you realize it or not, your environment, the movies you watch, the music you listen to, and the people around you all are influencing your daily thoughts. When you have a collection of thoughts about a particular thing, they become a belief. Have you ever had someone in your life that you may not have known personally but only ever heard negative things about them from other people, so you just believed it to be true? You finally meet the person and realize they are super nice, and all those preconceived beliefs about them were untrue.

The people around us, the media, social media, and various other outlets, a lot of times, can create beliefs in our minds that we accept as truth, which in reality, they couldn't be falser. This is why it's so important to guard your mind and your thoughts. You want to have thoughts that are reinforced by strong beliefs. This is why you need to be around people that will encourage, inspire, and empower you. People that will tell you, YOU CAN. You also need to tell yourself you can as well. The more positive reinforcement these beliefs get, the stronger they become. This is how you can develop a bulletproof mindset, and once that happens, it will positively influence the actions you take, which will lead to the results you desire. This is true in everything in life, whether it's a fitness goal, business, relationships, or anything else. Your better self and the life you desire first begins in your own mind.

Chapter 5

Iron Sharpens Iron

When you embark on a new journey, you may not have all the answers and may not always know what your next step should be, it is always a good idea to ask for help and guidance from people that you love and trust and also have been where you are. Many people, including myself many times, can be very stubborn and want to go about it alone. If you're going to go fast, go alone. But if you want to go far, go together. I can't stress enough how valuable it is to have mentors in your life that have traveled in your footsteps before and also to have good accountability partners. You should aim to have three types of people in your inner circle: mentors that have more experience than you that can teach and guide you, those on the same level as you where you can all hold each other accountable, and those that you can mentor. Why is the last one important? I believe you can learn a lot about yourself when you begin to mentor others. Part of successful leadership isn't just learning things on your own, but also being able to teach those lessons to others. Experience is the best teacher. But it doesn't always have to be YOUR experience.

My dad has been my biggest mentor, and I've learned many valuable lessons from him. I've learned many things I should do and things I should avoid based on his past experiences, not always my own. I'm a personal trainer and have worked with a lot of high school kids, and I view that as a time for me to not only help them physically but to be a "big bro" and mentor them. So, I receive mentorship, but I also mentor others who haven't yet been where I have been. If you want to learn something, teach it. I've found that to be one of the best ways to truly learn something. See someone do it first, then do it with them, then do it for someone else. That's how leadership should be. Just like iron sharpens iron, we must sharpen each other. Being a mentor to someone else will not only teach you a lot and help you personally, but it's also extremely fulfilling and rewarding and gives you a real sense of purpose. When you begin to do self-fulfilling things and you're giving back and making an impact, you're automatically going to be in a much better mood. If you're sad or depressed, do a good deed for someone else. I guarantee it'll make you feel a lot better. I've also noticed that when I give, I tend to receive even more. This isn't why I give, but it is a by-product of giving. I believe when you bless others, especially when you're in a difficult situation yourself, you will be blessed so much more. Being a servant and becoming more selfless truly can be an advantageous experience, and if you feel you lack purpose and fulfillment in your daily life, I promise you this will help change that. Impact someone else's life for the better and watch yours become much more blessed.

When you're seeking out a mentor, find someone that you trust that is where you want to be, or has what you want to have. Whether it's a marriage like theirs, a successful business like hers, a ripped physique like his, whatever the case may be, seek out people that are already there that can lead you there also. If you have never been to New York City before, you probably wouldn't ask someone who also has never been there for directions or what places you should see or what restaurants you should try. You would ask someone that goes there regularly or maybe lives there, right? This is how it should be with finding a good mentor. Someone that is where you want to be in life that is willing to help you. You can't pour from an empty cup, so find a full cup, let them pour their wisdom and experiences into you so that you can then pour into someone else. You don't want to repeat mistakes that others have made if you can help it. This can save you years of heartache, failures, money, and time. Be selective as to who you choose to mentor you, and allow them to hold you accountable. If you truly want better for yourself, allow someone to hold you to a higher standard. It's difficult to do this by yourself. Having support and accountability will take you to a much higher level so much quicker. The company you keep says a lot about you. Take a look at who you spend the most time with currently, whether it's family, friends, or co-workers. Do you feel they positively impact your life and environment? Some people and some relationships will be unavoidable but if they're toxic, keep your distance as much as possible, and surround yourself with more people that push and challenge you to be better and grow. You either influence your environment, or it will influence you. Become a better version of yourself so that you can positively influence those around you. A rising tide raises all ships. If you become better, you subconsciously invite others around you to become better too. Positivity, happiness, gratitude, and success can be very contagious, so surround yourself with those that have these qualities so that they may rub off on you, then you can share these gifts with others.

When I first got started on my entrepreneurial journey, I was waiting tables and had just graduated from college with a degree in Business. I always loved sales and commission-based opportunities where there was no ceiling on my income potential, and I could go out and get what I feel I'm worth. I got started in a network marketing company and surprisingly did pretty well right from the start. I ended up earning several thousand dollars a month and became one of the top producers in the company. So, I naturally decided to quit my table-waiting job and begin to pursue my networking business more full-time. Looking back, that wasn't one of my brightest moves. I had a good job and should've pursued both. Anytime you have multiple income streams, that's always a good place to be. I certainly wasn't "rich" by any means, but for someone that didn't have a "job" and at my age, I felt I was doing pretty well for myself and on my way to earning a substantial income in my early twenties.

Even though the future looked bright, and I was doing well for myself at the time, it was a struggle every day, and it was by no means easy. The only reason I did well in the beginning and finally started to get some momentum was because of my inner circle. Fortunately, I had family around me that supported me, even if they weren't involved in my business. They still loved me through it all, showed their support, and usually were always giving me referrals. I was also blessed to work with an amazing team that pushed me and challenged me constantly. I had people that mentored me, new people in the business that I mentored, and my close friends and partners that held me accountable. Had it not have been for the support and continued mentorship; I probably would not have lasted long. There's going to be many times along your journey, whether it's business, health, or just life where you will be faced with fear, uncertainty, and what seems like overwhelming self-doubt. There were many times I had doubt and thought, "Is this really something I can do?" I started to grow a huge team across multiple countries, and I was much younger at the time than mostly everyone in my team.

Many a times, I don't feel adequate enough and felt my age and lack of experience made me unfit to lead. It was something I battled for a long time. I didn't want to lead anyone astray; I wanted everyone to have success. I really wanted to believe that I was the leader that could lead them to the success they desired. But I wrestled with that. I thought, "Who am I to lead these people to massive financial wealth when I'm barely getting by myself?" There were times I was actually afraid of success. Sounds crazy, right? How could someone be afraid of succeeding? I knew that with great power comes great responsibility, and I feared being responsible for more people. Their families and livelihood depended on me and where I was leading them. I knew the more success I had, the more I would be traveling, mentoring, speaking on stage, and ultimately the more responsibility I would have. Even though these things excited me, they also did scare me because these were uncharted waters for me. I remember the first time I had to host a segment on stage in front of about 500 people. I was so nervous; I honestly thought I was going to throw up. I had spoken on stage many times, but now it was my turn to actually host an entire section. I used my "1, 2, 3, GO!" technique, started thinking about things I was grateful for, which immediately put me in a better mood, and I ran up to the stage to lead my segment. Fear and gratitude can't coexist. Remember that. I knew this was something I GET to do, not something

I HAVE to do. I'm blessed to be in the position to lead others. I'm blessed to receive this opportunity to be asked to present on stage and pour into others. Anytime you're in a position like this, it's also a chance for you to grow. Nothing grows in a comfort zone.

When you get uncomfortable like I was in that moment, you see what you're made of. You tap into another level and see that you truly are capable and that there's greatness within you. If you don't try, you'll never experience this side of you, and you'll never be able to share your gift with the world. Everyone has their unique song, and remember, only you can sing it. Like it says in Proverbs, "A man's gift makes room for him and brings him before great men..." I experienced many ups and downs with my network marketing business, and even though I have started other ventures and am involved in other opportunities, I'm still a part of that same community over six years later. My mentors and people that I met, whether through my team or someone else's, became some of my best friends and biggest supporters. Many of which I would consider my family. I've developed relationships and friendships with many of them, where I seek out guidance and support, even if it's not business-related. I can't stress enough how valuable this is for anyone looking to level-up in life. There are many people out there just like yourself that want better and are looking to improve areas in their own life. Once you embark on your journey to bettering yourself, it will open new doors and opportunities that will bring you to new relationships. I've left some friendships in the past that didn't serve me, and I've replaced a lot with friendships that force me to do and be better. It's not always personal or necessarily a bad thing. Still, sometimes you do need to be selfish and protect your energy and not allow anyone to steal away your joy or put negativity in your life. A happy and fulfilling life has no room for toxicity.

I would encourage you to try new things and intentionally put yourself in environments where there are other people just like yourself that are in the pursuit of "better." Go to a gym, or networking events, or a bible study. These can be great places to meet people that are seeking self-improvement. People with ambition and always seem to be happy and are just fun to be around; these are the people you want to have more of in your daily life. When I was younger, I joined a networking group that met every week. There were about 20 members from different industries, and these were some of the more successful and influential people in my area. I was just a young kid in my early twenties, but I was surrounding myself with ambitious bankers, real estate agents, lawyers, insurance brokers, business owners, and people of that nature. I wanted to level-up my circle and create a winning environment for myself.

You may be more of an introvert, and that's okay! Personally, many times I love being alone. As I'm writing this book, I currently live by myself, and I enjoy it, at least for now. I believe it's good to have a balance. Surround yourself with good people, and if you're more introverted, this is your opportunity to step outside of your comfort zone and allow yourself to grow. If you're someone that is constantly around people, it's also good to isolate yourself sometimes. Allow yourself time to think, pray, read, meditate, and get to know yourself. For me, this is when many ideas come to me, or when God may speak to you. It's good to be in silence at times. But have a balance, and when you are around others, be mindful and start to surround yourself with a winning circle. You want a strong starting-five if you ever want to win a championship.

Chapter 6

Defeating the Devil

As cliché as this may sound, I truly do believe everything happens for a reason. I believe if you look for the good in a person or situation, you'll find it. But the opposite is also true. If your brain is always programmed to see the negative, that's all you'll ever see and focus on, and as a result, more negative things will naturally be a part of your daily life because that's all that you notice. A glass of water that is half-full can either be viewed as half-full or half-empty. It's all perspective. Another example is, have you ever gone car shopping or maybe bought a new car and suddenly you start seeing that same make and model on the road a lot more frequently? Did the dealership just sell a bunch of those same cars that month, or were they always there, and you just never had a reason to notice them before? This is true about anything and everything in life. Five different people can all see the same movie, and all have different opinions about it. A lot of our perspectives and viewpoints today come from conditioning and programming from past experiences. Maybe things we were taught from our parents or school, or just experiences we went through. This shapes our existing reality. You may love Chick-fil-A, for example, but what if you went there and your chicken sandwich was terrible? You may think it was just a one-time unfortunate incident, but then you go back, and your next sandwich is terrible again. Your brain is now starting to correlate bad-tasting sandwiches with that particular place. We do the same with people, places, experiences, or anything in life. One bad experience can change our perspective forever, especially multiple bad experiences. Here's the good news. We can change this. This isn't super easy, nor will it ever be perfect; it will take practice. We must adopt the mindset that life is always happening FOR us, not TO us; we don't HAVE to do this, we GET to. I call this "flipping your filter." When you can see the good in every situation and person, your life immediately changes for the better.

One of the lowest points in my life was actually not too long ago. For a while, I was struggling financially, and that really wore on me mentally. My life in a lot of ways was not where it should be, and I knew it. I was wasting time and my God-given potential, which made me more depressed and unfulfilled. I was bouncing around from different side-gigs and odd-jobs. I was working in Richmond and commuting there every week and was planning on living there more permanently, so I sold my home. I was also still running a gym back home with my family. Even though I was working seven days a week, I wasn't super fulfilled with what I was doing and felt I should be in a much stronger place financially. After a few months of working in Richmond, I knew it wasn't going to be best for me long-term. I decide to come home and now basically being homeless, I had no other alternative at the moment but to move back in with my parents temporarily. But there was some light at the end of the tunnel, or so I thought… I finally got some good news after many strikeouts. Thanks to my mom and sister, I applied to be on a reality television show. After several months of silence, I received a phone call, which led to a Skype interview, then an interview in New York City, and eventually making it to the finalist week in Los Angeles. I was ready to go.

Things were finally looking up for me. I was beyond ready for a new adventure, new opportunity, and to meet some amazing new people. Then two weeks before leaving, I received a phone call, and was told they were going in a different direction and weren't going to bring me on this season. Bummer. It's easy to say, "well, everything happens for a reason," but at that moment, I had spent several months planning and was believing this was finally my time. A new start. A fresh beginning. In a new place. Ready for this new chapter. And just like that in a 6-minute phone call, that dream quickly faded. I ended up going out that weekend, which I rarely do. It was a fun night but ended with me spending the night in a cold, jail cell. Long story. Probably the worst night of my life. Two days later I get another call from a producer saying they decided they wanted to bring me on the show after all. Now, what do I do? It turned out I needed to fly to L.A. that night, or it pretty much wasn't in the cards for this season, and there was no way I could make that happen on such short notice. I was beyond honored and thrilled to have received such amazing news, but unfortunately, it couldn't have been worse timing for myself with filming starting in just three days, so I had to pass up the opportunity. Then the COVID-19 pandemic strikes. The entire world was on lockdown, and filming was postponed. It was a whirlwind of a week, let me tell you. I share this story with you to say this… it was a very dark time for me; I was very uncertain about the future and was at a crossroads. It would've been easy to just fold-up and complain and act like a victim, but I knew God was trying to teach me something. Good was going to come out of all this, and I was determined to see that through. You can't appreciate the sunny days if it never rains, but it's also hard to be grateful for a storm when you're still in it. I knew God had my back and I was already victorious; time just hadn't caught up yet.

During this period, I started to get very creative; I ended up launching a new business, created a new website, started an apparel line, began offering personal training services and coaching online, wrote an eBook, took a few online courses to learn some new skills, started auditioning for TV commercials, shows, movies, and app promos where I could do so remotely, and wrote this book. Had I not gone through what I did, none of this happens. I knew it happened exactly the way it needed to. We may have plans, but of course, they don't always go as planned. This is where faith comes in. You can't just throw in the towel. You may believe that your plans are good, but God wants better for you. Maybe that night doesn't happen, and maybe I actually make it on national television; would that have been better for me? I'll never know. But I do know God always has my best interest in mind; and when one door closes, another opens. You just need to trust Him and know you're in good hands. It was a dark time for me and one of my lowest, rock-bottom moments, but even in that jail cell, I knew God was testing me, and this was going to be part of my story that I would one day write about and share with the world.

We all face adversity, and what I've realized is it can be your downfall and worst enemy, or it can be your greatest fuel to propel you to new heights. I was down, but I knew that was another level with my name on it. I went through some crap, but I always knew God had a plan. We all deal with our struggles and problems in our own ways. I once had a mentor of mine tell me, "If we took all our problems and threw them into a big pile and saw everyone else's, we'd probably take ours back." My rock-bottom moment may not compare to someone that spent years in jail or someone that lost a loved one that was very close to them. But a rock-bottom moment for you is still a rock-bottom moment. There's no reason or benefit of comparing your lows and highs to someone else's because you don't honestly know what they're battling internally and what they've gone through. You may think spending one night in jail isn't so bad, and maybe it's not. It definitely could've been much worse. But that was a low point for me, especially with everything else going on in my life at that time; I was already in a valley of lows, and that was the icing on the cake. I knew I was going to bounce back but didn't know how to yet at that point. But I knew God was in control. Think about the athletes, authors, artists, musicians, actors, and people we look up to every day; people that we aspire to be like. You hear stories all the time of struggling actors or artists or musicians that overcome insane adversity, rejection, and failure.

This is why it's so important to be aligned with your true purpose and calling and also to have a very strong WHY. Something has to keep you going. Something has to keep pushing you when times are tough, to get you back on your feet when you fall. I call this failing forward. We all fall, but true failure is giving up. The struggling actor never quits, and eventually, he makes it on the big screen. Think about the story of Sylvester Stallone, a struggling actor that was so broke at one point, he had to sell his beloved dog and best friend just to afford food to survive. He later wrote the screenplay for Rocky and starred in it, and it became one of the most successful movies in

American history. Then, he went and bought his dog back. Everyone's journey is different and unique to them, so don't compare yours to someone else's. Don't compare your chapter 5 with someone else's chapter 20. Stay in your lane and focus on what you can control, and no matter what you want in life and whatever your purpose may be, the only true way to fail is to quit, so commit to yourself now that no matter what, you will not give up. The time will pass anyway, and there will be many setbacks, failures, heartache, and disappointments. But there will also be many victories, successes, and lives impacted if you never quit and follow the path God has laid out for you. Start to train your mind to see the good in every situation. I promise you if you look for it, you'll find it. You may not find it right away, but eventually, you will. Just like me, sitting in that jail cell. I knew good was going to come from it at some point. I didn't know when. But now here I am writing about it, sharing my story with you so hopefully, you don't make the same mistakes I made, and if it saves one life, it was all worth it. That's why you don't ever want to give up because your pain, adversity, and struggles could help someone else get out of the same mess you were in at one point. I knew God was going to turn my "mess" into my "message." There's nothing worse than a man who has been digging for gold for years and quits when he unknowingly was only 3 feet away from striking it. The point is, don't ever stop digging. Trust the process and embrace your journey, and you will change people's lives for the better. If enough of us do this, we create a ripple effect that can truly change the world.

Chapter 7

The "180."

I believe that one of the most selfless acts you can do is to actually become the very best possible version of yourself. You have gifts and talents and potential that you may have not even begun to scratch the surface of yet, which is true for most of us. When you "settle" in life, you're not giving the world your best. It should not only be a goal of ours, but our DUTY to become better in all areas of our life. I don't know about you, but I want to be the very best son, brother, friend, grandson, nephew, co-worker, and business partner I can be, and eventually, be the best dad and husband I can be. You owe it to your family or future family, your siblings, your parents, or your kids. Become the best YOU that you can be. It doesn't mean perfect. But the more you can do to improve yourself as a person and your situation, you will not only be bettering yourself but also those around you. You will start to subconsciously invite others to do the same, and you're just naturally going to have better relationships, friendships, and experiences altogether. I'm writing this book and sharing these stories with you to help you make that "180" in your own life, if it's necessary.

For you, maybe it's more of a physical and health journey; it may be more of a spiritual battle, or a tough financial situation. For me, it was a combination of many things, and I've learned if you neglect certain areas of your life and start to develop harmful habits, they will affect other areas of your life, which will also affect people around you. When you have constructive and positive habits and behaviors, you are going to be improving yourself as an individual, which will enhance your overall quality of life in all areas. You will then be encouraging those around you to start to embody their better selves. I believe we are called to have life and have it abundantly, and you can have that in this life. A life of happiness, fulfillment, joy, health, and abundance are available for all of us. It may seem too good to be true, but in these previous chapters, I have laid out for you steps that I took to help me get back on track and do a "180" in my own life. I'm by no means close to my ultimate goals, but the main thing is I know I'm heading in the right direction, and WOW does it feel so good to know you're in alignment with your true purpose! These strategies and principles will help get you on the path you're destined to be on. I'm not saying it will be easy and that these steps are going to take you to the Promised Land automatically, but they will help tremendously to improve everything in your life right now. Better mindset, better relationships, better finances, better health, a better body, a better walk with God, and just overall a better life. Focus on one day at a time, and know this is a journey of steps. You must be willing to take that first step and continuously step; it's a daily walk.

When I was in prep for my bodybuilding competition, in those final couple weeks, I was starting to break down mentally; physically, my body was extremely sore and never seemed to recover since I was training for up to three hours, seven days a week. But mentally, it was even worse. I was dreaming of food and felt I was always hungry, even though I was eating six meals per day. I couldn't get full, and I could only eat what those portions were and nothing more. It was quite torturous. So, I took it one day at a time. My goal was to "win" that day, not month or week, but simply be victorious one day at a time. I was counting down the days until it was all over so I could at least eat a piece of bread for goodness sake! Being three weeks out felt like three years, but I knew I just had to attack it one day at a time, one meal at a time, one workout at a time. The same is true in business or our lives. Focus on .01% improvement each day. You will have days you don't feel like doing anything and days where you feel like you're failing and losing the race; it's all part of the process! That's why I said in the last chapter to expect this, but never stop digging. Have something in front of you that you're chasing. It might be something you're looking forward to, a goal you're trying to achieve, or whatever the case may be. For me, it was stepping on that stage in as good of shape as possible.

When you have that in front of you, it tends to PULL you. If you constantly push yourself, you may burnout; but if the vision and the ultimate goal is strong enough, it will pull you towards it like a magnet. It's like running a marathon; halfway through you feel exhausted and may want to quit, but you take another step, then another. Then you see the finish line and suddenly get this newfound burst of energy to finish strong. Keep your "finish line" in sight so that it pulls you towards it constantly. Of course, in life, there is no ultimate "finish line," but whatever that is for you as far as a short-term goal or life-long vision, keep it in the forefront of your mind always and allow it to pull you. Understand your journey isn't about perfection, but rather consistency. That's why habits are so important. Habits will lead you to your wildest dreams, or they will destroy you. I've had some destructive habits in my own life that I had to first acknowledge that they existed and that they didn't serve me, and then take baby-steps to "turn" those habits around for the better. If you can develop healthy, productive habits in your life and have people around you to help hold you accountable, you, my friend, are well on your way to a much happier, healthier, and fulfilled life.

A philosophy I adopted years ago was to make each year of my life better than the previous year. I've had many older adults tell me the "college years" are the best of your life. How sad is that? I never bought into that bogus lie. College was fun for me, but after I graduated, I began my entrepreneurial journey and started traveling, meeting all sorts of amazing people, and having crazy life experiences. It wasn't all peaks, though. There were a lot of valleys. My twenties have been a roller-coaster, but I can honestly say my life has gradually gotten better each year since college; so good news for you if you're still in college, just graduated, or maybe haven't started yet. Really, it's still good news no matter what your age is. This is a philosophy you can adopt right now, and understand your life journey is YOURS and yours only. Colonel Sanders was 62 years old when he started Kentucky Fried Chicken. Ray Kroc was in his mid-50's when he bought his first McDonald's. Morgan Freeman was in his 40's when he caught his first big break. The point is age doesn't matter. As I'm writing this, I'm currently 28 years old.

I may be behind a lot of 28-year-olds right now, but in 2 years, I believe I will be light-years ahead of most 30-year-olds. That's how you have to think. It's not about comparing yourself to others, but realizing that you have to start at some point if you want BETTER, and you have to focus on competing with no one other than yourself. This isn't a race; it's about becoming a better YOU. Tony Robbins said, "People may overestimate what they can accomplish in 1 year, but severely underestimate what they can do in 10." Think about that for a second. It's easy at the start of the new year to set these big, lofty goals that we may never achieve that year. But how many of us set goals 5, 10, or more years down the road? Let's say you're reading this right now, and you're only 37 years old. You may or may not be happy with your current lifestyle and position, and that's okay; ten years is a long time. It goes fast, but think about what all you can accomplish in ten years… That makes you only 47-years-old. Still very young in the big scheme of life. You may not be the most successful 40-year-old, but you can become much more successful than most

50-year-olds. That's the type of mindset you want to develop.

Each year of your life, strive to make it better than the previous in all areas! I focus on being 1% better each year, each month, each day. If you do this, your life has no choice but to improve every day and every year forward. Focus on one day at a time. How do you eat an elephant? One bite at a time.

It's worth noting too that while we're all on this journey of "better," to also enjoy the process. I truly believe happiness is a CHOICE. It's not a side-effect of something happening, although it could be. Happiness is something that you can choose to be every moment of every day. It's not always super easy, but it certainly is possible. Especially when you live with an attitude of gratitude. When you are grateful, it will make you happy; you can't be sad or upset when you're in a state of gratitude. There's so much we all take for granted on a daily basis, and none of us is promised tomorrow. A couple of months ago was the death of N.B.A. legend, Kobe Bryant. Growing up watching him play, I could've sworn he was a real-life superhero. He seemed invincible, and just like that in a horrific helicopter crash, his life was gone in an instant. It seemed the entire world paused for a moment. He was a global icon that was just beginning his retirement from basketball and starting his entrepreneurial career. I think we all viewed him and people like him as immortal, and for this terrible incident to occur, it made us all realize how precious and vulnerable life is and that we are all human. Then several weeks later, the COVID-19 outbreak happens, putting most of the world on complete lockdown, taking away everyday things that we take for granted. Something as simple as a handshake, a hug, going to grab some lunch with a friend, taking your significant other out for ice cream, or taking a date to the movies all suddenly came to an abrupt halt. In these times, I try to be mindful of how short, precious, and fragile life is. Like my Papa used to say, "Life is just a look out the window;" so be happy, choose happiness, every day, and be present in each moment. I don't always do this, but I try to be intentional when I am with someone or maybe in a place I've never been before. I want to take it in and absorb it fully; embrace every moment because this time is precious.

Chapter 8

All In

In today's society, there are so many distractions. With technology advancing as quickly as it is, we now have phones that are more intelligent than we are. Our phones today are literally small computers, and we have the ability to use them for just about everything, not just phone calls. Whether you want to bank online, pay your bills, watch videos, read, start a business, create content, take photos, invest in stocks, do video chats, online dating, and the list goes on. Anything you can think of, there's most likely an app for that. Just on our cellphones, there are unlimited distractions, and it's something most of us carry around with us 24/7. I know this feeling all too well as I run all my businesses and pretty much my entire life through my phone. It can be a great tool, but also a massive distraction. I've noticed personally that when I get laser-focused on a task and minimize distractions, I am much more productive. I use our phones as an example, but anything can be a distraction. It could be your TV or the radio or even certain toxic people in your life. When I have my best results, it's always when I limit my distractions to the best of my ability and set a deadline for whatever it is that I'm working on or towards. You've made it this far in this book, so I assume you're serious about making changes to truly better yourself. It's time now to make the decision and go ALL IN and fully commit to YOURSELF. Nothing changes if nothing changes. "Insanity" is doing the same thing repeatedly over and over again but expecting a different result. You know if you want to make your situation better, whatever it may be, it's going to require change, growth, adaptation, and being able to overcome. It won't always be easy, but it's always worth it.

For myself, many times I know that I can be a very "A.D.H.D." type person, and even though it was a lot worse for me when I was younger, I still deal with this today; and truthfully with as many messages and ads that we're exposed to daily, we probably all somewhat are. I have learned from this and had to make adjustments accordingly to maximize my time and minimize distractions. It's also taught me to manage my time more effectively and efficiently. However, when I am working on a project, I tend to go ALL IN and get laser-focused on that specific thing I'm working on until it's complete. Our attention spans are very short, and I know mine is for sure, so I usually block out about 90 minutes or so of intentional, laser-focused work. Then I have to take a break because I can tell my productivity and focus starts to gradually decline after that amount of time. I usually try to work out or do something physical if I can just to move my body, then I'll go back to work. This is what suits me best and allows me to be the most productive. Even though at times my mind seems to be all over the place, I've been able to use this to my benefit, and when I hone in on a task or goal, I get obsessive with it until it's finished, whether it was playing basketball in high school, getting into bodybuilding in college, or starting into entrepreneurship, I always tend to go all in. I share this with you because there are probably things in your life that aren't perfect or things you deal with that will interfere with your commitment and your goals.

It could be a physical or mental disability or anything that can hinder your progress, but I'm here to tell you that you can use it to your advantage if you get creative enough. I know how A.D.D. I can be, so for me to write a book almost seemed like something that was going to be impossible for me. It takes me a while to read a book, let alone write one. But just like with anything in life, I've learned to discipline myself. I force myself to read because I know it's good for me and will force me to grow. Also, like I am forcing myself to write a little bit each day until this book is done. Remember, when I shared with you earlier about seeking some type of discomfort daily? I'm not always in the mood to read, but I force myself to do it anyway. Just like with working out; don't work out just when you feel motivated because motivation is temporary. Force and discipline yourself to stick with a schedule. If you commit to reading ten pages a day and working out three days a week, then do it. Of course, if you don't, no one will ever know, but you'll know, and you'll know you're just cheating yourself out of the better life you want and deserve. There may be obstacles or roadblocks in your life, whether they're real or just in your head, but don't let that stop you. It may slow you down, but get creative and adapt. Seek counsel if necessary, but I'm telling you whatever you may be dealing with could be fuel to your fire. Turn your imperfections into weapons; own them, and use them to further yourself. It took me a few years to understand how I operated and how to use it to my benefit. I can be easily distracted; therefore, I have to try extra hard to limit my distractions so I can be more productive, but I know once I set my sights on something, I'll obsess over it until it's complete. This may not be the best method for you, but I've found that's how I can operate at a higher level for me personally. Understand yourself and how you tick; are you more productive in the morning or at night? There's no right or wrong way, but there are ways that can be much more beneficial for your lifestyle and your goals long-term. Once you learn yourself, you can manage your time and develop your routines so that they can be optimized and most efficient as possible. Whether you work out consistently or not, I would strongly encourage you to at least move your body as much as possible throughout the week. I know people that get their workout in at 5 A.M. because they know after work, they'll be too tired. Everyone's schedules are different. You just need to find what suits you best.

Remember, this is going to be an ongoing process, and everything isn't just going to happen overnight. Start by maybe waking up 30 minutes earlier each day, and use that 30 minutes to stretch, meditate, pray, read, journal, or do yoga. Try it; you have nothing to lose, and you'll be surprised what other creative and productive ideas that'll spark. Create a routine that you fall in love with that's productive and serves you, and one that you can't wait to get up the next morning to do again. This is how you can achieve success in all areas of your life over time. The key to success lies in your daily routine.

Life will pay whatever price you ask of it; so be careful what you ask. Even if you feel you're not "asking" anything, you actually are. The world awaits to hear your story; no one else can sing your song. There have been many times in my life I shared a story or experience with someone that unknowingly was going through something similar and ended up having a massive impact on their life. When you stay silent, you could be missing out on helping someone and also receiving blessings for yourself by doing so. You don't know the ripple effect that can be created by you sharing your story with one person; maybe it's one Facebook post, or perhaps it's one text message to a friend. You never know what someone may be dealing with on the inside, so never be afraid to share your story with others.

One of my favorite stories is the Parable of the Talents, as told in the Bible. If you're not familiar with the story, I'll briefly summarize it. There was a rich ruler that went away on business and left his three servants talents based on their respective abilities. A talent was a sum of money, although some believe this parable was about our actual talents and God-given gifts. Regardless of the message, the principles are the same. He gave five talents to one servant, two to another, and one to the third. The servant with five talents went out and doubled his master's investment and got five more, now totaling ten. The servant with two did the same and went out and produced two more, now totaling four, but the servant with one talent went and buried his and hid it in fear of losing it. When the master returned from his voyage, the servant with ten talents showed him that he doubled his investment, and the master was so proud—the same with the servant with four talents. When the servant with one talent told the master what he had done, the master called him lazy and took his one talent and gave it to the servant who had ten. If you are faithful with little things, you will be faithful with larger things. But if you can't be trusted with little things, you won't be entrusted with greater responsibilities. I believe this parable has a lot of financial truth to it and can be interpreted on a few different levels. One of my biggest takeaways is the servant who had been given a talent and did nothing with it. There are so many people today that have been given "talents," whether it was 1, 5, or 100 that are choosing to "bury" and "hide" them rather than to invest them and allow God to multiply them. To whom much is given, much will be required. I've learned not to pray for a lighter load, but that God would give me stronger shoulders. He'll never give you more than you can handle. Trust that. So whatever you're dealing with currently, know that you have what it takes to overcome.

Everything is temporary; when life is good, cherish it, and fully receive it. When life is bad, remember that it won't last, and better days arc ahead. Note also that it doesn't matter who has the most or least talents; we are given talents based on what the master decides; so, it's not about how many you have, but rather what will you do with the ones you have now? Use them? Multiple them? Hide them? Another takeaway from the lazy servant is he was fearful. He didn't even TRY to invest his master's money; he just took it and hid it to protect it, but that's not really what the master wanted. This is also true in our lives. It's not about how much you can do and produce, but rather having faith and not being fearful and trusting in your talents to go out and make the most of them. We don't always have control of the outcome, but we do have control over our actions, so focus on what you CAN control and leave the rest up to God; this will bring about much peace if you can live your life this way.

One of my biggest fears in life is regret. I think that's one of the things I probably think about the most. I look at my life right now, and I think, "Am I really using my talents as I should be? Am I maximizing my potential? Do I have any talents that I have buried and hidden?" These questions truly haunt me at times. I don't want to be at the end of my life and look back and hate myself for not simply TRYING; for not going after that dream. For, in the end, it's not the things we did, but the things we didn't do and opportunities and experiences missed that we will regret; so take the shot! You'll never know what it feels like to hit a game-winning

3-pointer if you never shoot, or a walk-off homer in the bottom of the 9th if you never swing. Sure, you'll miss, and you'll strikeout a ton as I have; but I know with each strikeout, I'm that much closer to a grand slam. What separates the master from the servant? The master has failed more times than the servant has even tried. I'm not saying all this now to hype you up and try and motivate you. At this point, I hope deep down you recognize some areas that maybe need some attention in your life and are now ready and willing to finally "get up off the nail" and pursue the life you're destined to live.

Something else to keep in mind is the power of your thoughts. You will become what you continuously tell yourself and think about. I know we talked about this earlier, but it's worth mentioning again. You have all the tools necessary to win, and WIN BIG! You will have support along the way, but you'll also have naysayers and people that will judge, criticize, and condemn you no matter what you do.

But you really only need one person to believe in you; one person to tell you that YOU CAN, and that's YOU. This is your life, your destiny, your calling, your purpose; don't take those talents and unfulfilled dreams and promises to the grave with you. We are in a time and place now where the world truly needs good leaders and role models. Your story needs to be shared, and for some extra encouragement, just know that I have wanted to write a book for years, and I kept putting it off thinking to myself, "Who am I to write a book? I'm just a kid. No one will read it." But I finally had to silence the voices in my head and all the self-doubt and say, "I AM WORTHY" and the time is "NOW."

My story may be far different than yours; not better or worse, just different, but there are many lives I may not be able to reach that you can. You have a song that I can't sing, so that's why I'm telling you to be brave enough to share it. You may not always feel like it, but again remember, this life isn't meant to always be comfortable. If you want improvement and success in any area of your life, it will take sacrifice and discipline, but it's always worth it. Even if not for you, do it for your family or future family.

Don't hide your talents; go out and use them, invest them, multiply them, and make your master proud. The further you go, the further you'll see. As I mentioned earlier, motion creates emotion; you're not always going to feel "motivated" or "inspired," but you must learn to discipline those feelings and move anyway. Once you move, you'll begin to tap into personal momentum. If you lay around and do nothing and wait for that spark of inspiration, you may be waiting a long time. Learn to move despite what you're feeling and tap into your momentum, just like the shark that keeps swimming so it doesn't drown; you must also keep moving. The results you'll start to see will become addicting, which will fuel even more movement. The key is to begin and don't worry about how you "feel" or wait for that "perfect time." NOW is the perfect time.

I want to thank you for supporting me and taking the time to read some of my story. At times even though I still feel like a kid, I have been through a lot at my age, and I felt it was time to share my story. If one person reads this and it changes their life for the better, or maybe it encourages them to share their story, which then causes a positive ripple effect, it was all worth it to me. I'm not writing this book by accident or doing it because I'm just bored; I'm doing it because I believe there are people out there hurting and suffering and feel that they'll never be good enough to really make an impact in the world. I want to show them that their life matters and they are not here by accident! I want you to discover your purpose in this life and to start living for something much bigger than just yourself. If life was just about us, then really, what is the point of it?

We are destined for so much more. We are part of a bigger and greater plan. We have greatness within us; we just first need to believe in ourselves. Like in the parable, some people have five talents, or two, or maybe just one. But again, it doesn't matter who has what. What matters is what YOU have and what you do with it. Whether you have one talent or 100. You will be judged according to what God gave you and you alone. After finishing this book, take some alone time for yourself. You may or may not journal, but I would encourage you just to write down your thoughts and truly start to soul-search. Be REAL with yourself, and focus on some areas in your life that you truly wish were better.

Maybe your health, your finances, your relationship with your kids or parents, your spiritual journey, or maybe a combination of all of these. Write them down and ask yourself those questions we discussed earlier on. "Who am I? What do I love? What do I hate? What makes me weep?" Begin to search your soul and ask for God's guidance and to give you peace and clarity. The foundation begins by you acknowledging the areas that need improvement. Once we know what to focus on, we can begin to develop the right activities and behaviors to help make these goals our new reality. For example, say we want to lose a few pounds. So how are we doing to do this? First, we acknowledge what it is that we want to change. We write down our goals and give them a deadline. I want to lose 8 pounds in the next 30 days, let's say. Okay great! Now what?

We need a plan of action. We need to commit to it and start small and grow from there. If we aren't doing anything physically currently, let's start with two times per week we're going to walk or at least move our body. Next week we'll do three times and maybe add an extra 10-15 minutes onto each session. It may not seem like much, but progress is progress. Even if it's just a tiny bit, remember, you're either going forward or backward in life. There is no standstill; forward is still forward, whether it's a giant leap or a baby-step. Also, remember that if nothing changes, nothing changes, so we need to tweak your routine. You might be super busy, but what is something we can sacrifice that would free up some time for you? If you watch 2 hours of TV a night, could you reduce it to 90 minutes and then have 30 minutes free to exercise? You'll need to get creative. That is if you want BETTER, of course. Get a routine set and share it with someone. Maybe you even walk or workout with someone. Have an accountability partner. Or even hire a trainer if you need to. There are many times I'll send someone a text or message just to check in with them and their health goals, even if they're not my client and never paid me for my services; I just want to help them see results. And I also know the power that one simple text can have on someone. People like to be congratulated, encouraged, and patted on the back, so I'm always more than willing to help push someone along the right path. This isn't all going to happen overnight; each day, try and move in that direction. Eventually you'll develop that "winner's routine," and your mindset will become more "bulletproof," but it begins with a DECISION. Draw a line in the sand, commit to yourself, burn those boats, and don't look back! Your past is in the past, leave it there and focus on the here and now, and where you are heading. It will take time, but you'll get there. Remember, the time will pass anyway, so you might as well start now moving in the direction you want to go. Ten years from now, you could have a dream life and look back and be so grateful that you took the necessary steps today so that you and your family could have a better tomorrow. From this point forward, make the declaration that each year of your life will be better than the previous, and YOUR BEST IS YET TO COME!

Once you acknowledge the areas in your life that you want to focus on improving, write down your goals and make them visible so that you see them every day, even multiple times a day. Keep them in sight, and share them with someone else if you'd like. This part you may not do, but I can tell you from experience that your success rate with anything in life will skyrocket when you have solid people around you holding you accountable to your goals, especially if they are to be done by a certain deadline. Always put a time-stamp on your goals, otherwise, it's easy to get lazy and procrastinate and just put them on the back-burner. Start to exercise your mind, as well. Reading and journaling is great, but be very careful what you feed your mind daily. Every thought you think and word you speak has incredible power. Be careful what you say about yourself because you are always listening, and be careful what you think about yourself because thoughts do become things. If you're struggling in an area, write it down. Writing helps to address the actual problem and gets your creative mind working to find a solution to it. Feed your mind positivity as much as possible. I love movies and music, but I do try and be mindful of what I am constantly feeding my brain. Garbage in, garbage out. This is why when I drive or work out sometimes, I'll listen to podcasts, or if I'm walking on the stair-master doing cardio, I may put on a YouTube video of something inspiring or someone that motivates me. It's fun to watch Netflix every once in a while, but try and be mindful of what your subconscious mind is consuming and how much it's consuming daily. If you're going to watch something, try a documentary, or anything that'll stretch your mind and maybe spark some creativity. You may have a super busy schedule, but I would also encourage you to find some hobbies you enjoy. Preferably one that makes you money, one that keeps you in shape, or one that you just simply love doing and is therapeutic for you. I have found for myself that if I stay busy with a project, it keeps me out of trouble. When I'm bored at times, it's much easier to watch TV or cheat on your diet or do things that could potentially set you back on your goals. Nothing is wrong with these things, but I just want you to be aware of where your time goes and how many things daily do you do simply because they feel good, but maybe don't bring about any real value to your life that will support your future self. When you become aware of these things, you can now take action steps to make some changes.

I want you to start small, but the key is to START! Take it one day at a time, and focus on winning that day. It's not easy to turn a cruise ship around. It takes time and massive energy for a ship to do a complete "180." The same is true for us. The good news is it is, in fact, possible! But it's also true that it will indeed take some time. You will have highs with the lows, and go through rock-bottom type moments as I did. Your low point isn't your downfall; it can be a platform that springs you to new and greater heights. I know if it weren't for the lows in my life, I wouldn't be writing this book right now. It's because of my failures, setbacks, missed opportunities, and losses, that is the reason I am here today, and I'm now sharing my experiences with you. What are some things in your life or rock-bottom moments that you went through or are currently going through that can be used as a platform for good? Use your adversity as fuel. This is how you defeat the devil. He can't win if every time he knocks you down, you get back up. You got this. Your best is yet to come. Make each year of your life from this point forward better than the previous one. Focus on growth, and focus forward. You either WIN or you LEARN; there is no losing. There is no quitting; not this time. Your quest for "better" has begun. I look forward to seeing your growth and the many lives that will be impacted because of it.

Here's to BETTER!
Your Friend,
Mikey B.